# Diabetic Renal Diet Cookbook for Beginners

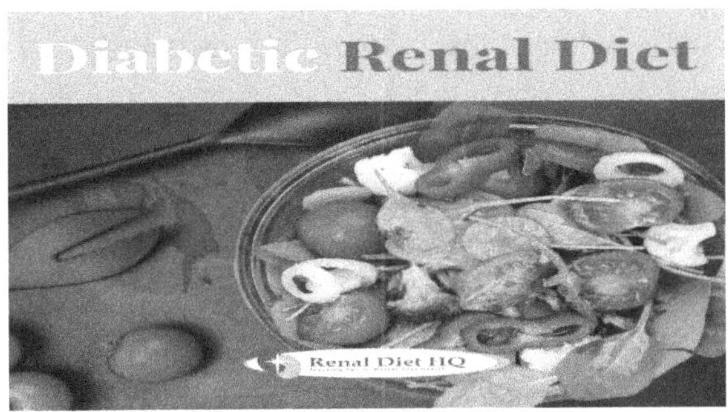

Easy Guide to Low Sodium, Low Potassium, Low Phosphorus, Low Sugar, Low Carb and Delicious Foods for an Overall Health and Well-being

Isaac Hendricks

# Table of Contents

# INTRODUCTION

## Understanding Diabetic Renal Diets

### Overview of Diabetes and Renal Health

Managing diabetes and renal health is a crucial aspect of overall well-being, requiring a nuanced understanding of the intricate relationship between these two conditions. Diabetes, a metabolic disorder characterised by elevated blood sugar levels, can significantly impact kidney function over time, leading to diabetic nephropathy or renal complications.

### The Connection Between Diabetes and Renal Health:

- Diabetes and the Kidneys: Explore how prolonged high blood sugar levels can strain the kidneys, affecting their ability to filter waste and excess fluids.

- Risk Factors: Understand the factors that increase the likelihood of diabetic nephropathy, including genetics, blood pressure, and duration of diabetes.

Impact on Kidney Function:

- Microvascular Changes: Examine the microvascular changes in the kidneys due to diabetes, leading to alterations in glomerular filtration and renal blood flow.

- Albuminuria: Learn about the significance of albuminuria, a key marker of kidney damage in individuals with diabetes.

Importance of Nutrition in Managing Diabetes and Renal Concerns:

- Dietary Guidelines: Explore the role of a well-balanced diet in managing diabetes and supporting renal health.

- Nutrient Monitoring: Understand the importance of monitoring nutrients like sodium, potassium, and phosphorus to alleviate strain on the kidneys.

Lifestyle Modifications:

- Physical Activity: Discuss the positive impact of regular physical activity in controlling blood sugar levels and maintaining overall health.

- Blood Pressure Management: Highlight the importance of blood pressure control in preventing further damage to the kidneys.

- Healthcare Team: Emphasise the significance of a collaborative approach involving healthcare professionals, nutritionists, and individuals in managing diabetes and renal health.

- Patient Empowerment: Encourage individuals to take an active role in their health by making informed lifestyle choices and adhering to prescribed treatments.

Understanding the intricate interplay between diabetes and renal health lays the foundation for proactive management, empowering individuals to adopt lifestyle modifications and dietary choices that promote overall well-being. This overview serves as a guide for navigating the complexities of these conditions and fostering a holistic approach to health maintenance.

## Importance of Nutrition in Managing Diabetes and Renal Concerns

The significance of nutrition in managing diabetes and renal concerns cannot be overstated, as dietary choices play a pivotal role in supporting overall health and mitigating the progression of these conditions. A carefully tailored diet can help regulate blood sugar levels, alleviate stress on the kidneys, and enhance overall well-being. Here's why nutrition is crucial in navigating the intricate relationship between diabetes and renal health:

### Blood Sugar Control:

**Carbohydrate Management:** Proper nutrition involves monitoring and balancing carbohydrate intake to prevent spikes in blood sugar levels.

**Glycemic Index Awareness:** Emphasising foods with a low glycemic index aids in better blood sugar control, promoting stable energy levels.

### Renal-Friendly Nutrient Monitoring:

**Sodium Restriction:** Managing sodium intake is essential to control blood pressure and reduce fluid retention, easing the workload on the kidneys.

**Potassium and Phosphorus Balance:** Monitoring and adjusting potassium and phosphorus intake helps prevent imbalances that can impact kidney function.

### Protein Moderation:

**Controlled Protein Intake:** Balancing protein consumption is vital to reduce the strain on the kidneys, as excessive protein can exacerbate renal issues.

**High-Quality Protein Sources:** Opting for lean and high-quality protein sources supports muscle health without compromising kidney function.

**Fluid Balance:** Maintaining proper hydration is crucial for kidney function and helps prevent dehydration-related complications.

**Limiting Sugary Drinks:** Choosing water over sugary beverages supports hydration without contributing to blood sugar fluctuations.



**Antioxidant-Rich Foods:** Incorporating fruits and vegetables rich in antioxidants helps combat inflammation and oxidative stress associated with diabetes and renal concerns.

**Essential Vitamins and Minerals:** Ensuring an adequate intake of vitamins and minerals supports overall health and immune function.



**Individualised Approach:** Recognizing that nutritional needs vary, personalised dietary plans can be crafted in collaboration with healthcare professionals, considering factors such as age, weight, and specific health conditions.

**Continuous Monitoring and Adjustments:** Regular assessment and adjustments to dietary plans enable individuals to adapt to changing health needs over time.

Adopting a nutritionally mindful approach is a cornerstone in the management of diabetes and renal concerns. By making informed dietary choices, individuals can enhance their quality of life, reduce the risk of complications, and actively contribute to their overall health and well-being.

# CHAPTER ONE

## Building a Foundation

### Kitchen Essentials for Diabetic Renal Cooking

Creating a diabetic renal-friendly kitchen involves equipping yourself with the right tools and ingredients to make wholesome and balanced meals that support both diabetes management and kidney health. Here are essential items for your kitchen:

**1. Measuring Tools:**
   - Accurate measurements are crucial for managing portion sizes and monitoring nutrient intake. Invest in measuring cups and spoons for precision in ingredient quantities.

**2. Nonstick Cookware:**
   - Nonstick pans reduce the need for excessive cooking oils, promoting heart health and supporting weight management.

**3. Food Scale:**
   - A food scale assists in portion control, helping you manage carbohydrate and protein intake effectively.

### 4. Slow Cooker or Instant Pot:

   - These appliances make it easy to prepare nutritious and flavorful meals with minimal added fats and salts.

### 5. Cutting Boards and Sharp Knives:

   - High-quality cutting boards and sharp knives simplify the preparation of fresh fruits, vegetables, and lean proteins.

### 6. Low-Sodium Seasonings:

   - Enhance flavours without compromising kidney health by using herbs, spices, and low-sodium seasonings instead of excessive salt.

### 7. Steamer Basket:

   - Steaming is a healthy cooking method that retains the nutritional value of vegetables while requiring minimal added fats.

### 8. Nutrient-Dense Ingredients:

   - Stock your pantry with nutrient-dense options like whole grains, legumes, lean proteins, and a variety of colourful fruits and vegetables.

### 9. Low-Glycemic Sweeteners:

   - Opt for alternatives to refined sugars, such as stevia or monk fruit, to sweeten recipes without causing spikes in blood sugar.

### 10. Kidney-Friendly Proteins:

- Include sources of high-quality protein such as fish, poultry, tofu, and legumes to support muscle health and minimise stress on the kidneys.

## 11. Nonperishable Staples:
   - Keep a supply of nonperishable items like canned tomatoes, low-sodium broths, and whole-grain pasta for convenient, kidney-conscious meals.

## 12. Water Filtration System:
   - Staying hydrated is crucial for kidney health. A water filtration system ensures access to clean, safe water without added impurities.

## 13. Label Reading Skills:
   - Develop the habit of reading food labels to identify hidden sugars, sodium, and phosphorus content in packaged items.

## 14. Storage Containers:
   - Invest in a variety of storage containers for portioning and storing leftovers, making it easier to adhere to recommended serving sizes.

By assembling these kitchen essentials, you create a supportive environment for preparing diabetic renal-friendly meals. Adopting a mindful and informed approach to cooking contributes to the overall well-being of individuals managing both diabetes and renal health.

# Grocery Shopping Tips and Ingredient Substitutions

Navigating the grocery store with a focus on diabetic renal-friendly ingredients requires careful planning and awareness. Consider these tips to make your shopping experience more efficient and health-conscious:

## 1. Plan Ahead:

- Create a weekly meal plan and corresponding shopping list to ensure you have all the necessary ingredients for balanced and kidney-friendly meals.

## 2. Stick to the Perimeter:

- The perimeter of the grocery store typically contains fresh produce, lean proteins, and dairy—optimal choices for a diabetic renal diet.

## 3. Choose Fresh Produce:

- Prioritise fresh fruits and vegetables, but be mindful of potassium content. Opt for lower-potassium options such as berries, apples, and cauliflower.

## 4. Read Labels Carefully:

- Scrutinise food labels for sodium, sugar, and phosphorus content. Choose low-sodium and low-sugar options whenever possible.

## 5. Opt for Whole Grains:

   - Select whole grains like quinoa, brown rice, and whole wheat bread over refined grains to enhance fibre content and manage blood sugar levels.

## 6. Lean Proteins:

   - Include sources of lean protein such as skinless poultry, fish, tofu, and legumes. Limit processed meats and high-fat cuts.

## 7. Low-Fat Dairy:

   - Choose low-fat or fat-free dairy products to maintain healthy fat levels and support kidney function.

## 8. Mindful Snacking:

   - Look for diabetic renal-friendly snacks like nuts, seeds, and fresh fruits. Avoid processed snacks high in sodium and sugar.

## 9. Experiment with Herbs and Spices:

   - Build a collection of kidney-friendly herbs and spices to add flavour without relying on excess salt.

## 10. Hydration Choices:

   - Opt for water, herbal teas, or low-sugar beverages to stay hydrated. Minimise the intake of sugary drinks and limit caffeine if advised.

## 1. Salt Alternatives:
- Substitute salt with herbs, spices, and vinegar to enhance flavour without compromising on kidney health.

## 2. Sugar Alternatives:
- Replace refined sugars with natural sweeteners like stevia, monk fruit, or erythritol to manage blood sugar levels.

## 3. Whole Grain Swaps:
- Swap refined grains with whole grains like quinoa, bulgur, or barley for increased fibre and better blood sugar control.

## 4. Lean Protein Choices:
- Opt for lean protein sources such as skinless poultry, fish, tofu, and legumes instead of high-fat or processed meats.

## 5. Low-Potassium Options:
- Choose lower-potassium fruits and vegetables, such as apples, berries, cabbage, and green beans, to regulate potassium intake.

## 6. Portion Control:
- Use smaller plates and bowls to naturally control portion sizes and avoid overeating.

By incorporating these grocery shopping tips and ingredient substitutions into your routine, you can empower yourself to make informed choices that align with a diabetic renal-friendly lifestyle. This mindful approach to shopping and cooking is essential for supporting overall health and well-being.

# LOW PROTEIN FOOD

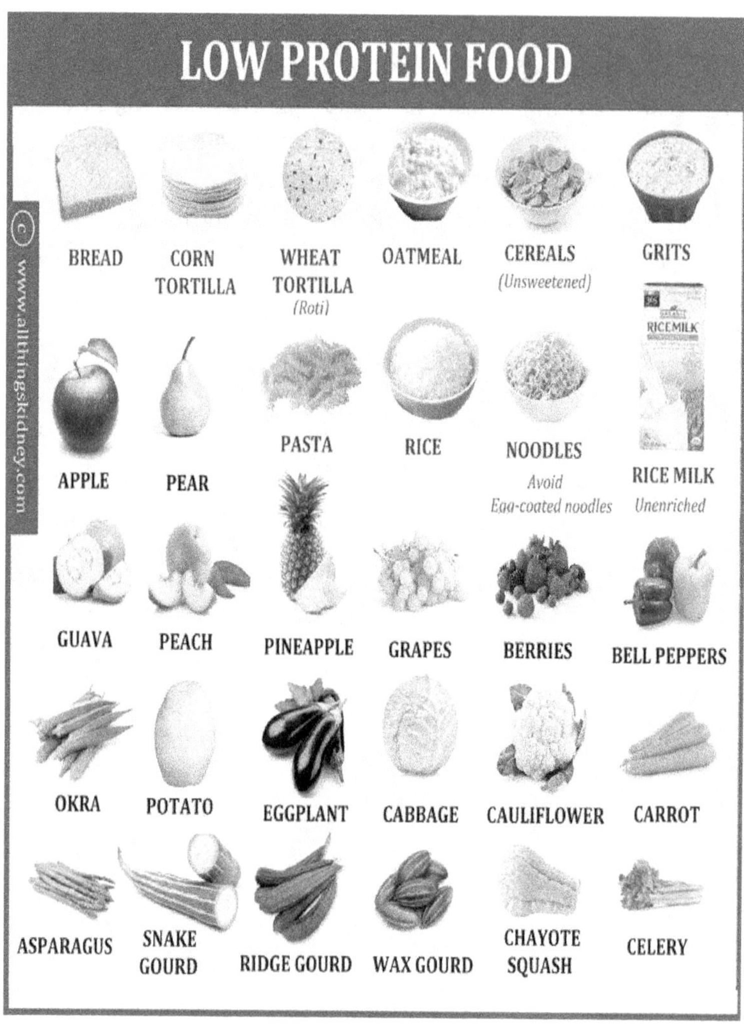

# CHAPTER TWO

## Breakfast Delights

### Berry Blast Oatmeal Bowl

Berry Blast Oatmeal Bowl is a delicious and nutritious breakfast option for those following a diabetic renal diet. This recipe is perfect for beginners as it is easy to prepare and packed with essential nutrients that are beneficial for people with diabetes and kidney disease.

**Ingredients:**
- 1/2 cup rolled oats
- 1 cup unsweetened almond milk
- 1/2 cup frozen mixed berries
- 1 tablespoon chia seeds
- 1 tablespoon ground flaxseed
- 1 tablespoon honey (optional)
- 1/4 teaspoon cinnamon
- 1/4 teaspoon vanilla extract

**Instructions:**
1. In a medium saucepan, combine the rolled oats, unsweetened almond milk, frozen mixed berries, chia seeds, ground flaxseed, honey (if desired), cinnamon, and vanilla extract. Stir well to combine.
2. Cook the oatmeal over medium heat, stirring occasionally, until it reaches your desired consistency. This should take about 5-7 minutes.

3. Once the oatmeal is cooked, remove it from the heat and let it cool for a few minutes before serving.
4. Divide the oatmeal into two bowls and serve immediately.
5. Garnish with additional berries and a sprinkle of cinnamon, if desired.

This Berry Blast Oatmeal Bowl is not only delicious but also packed with essential nutrients that are beneficial for people with diabetes and kidney disease. Rolled oats are a good source of fibre, which can help regulate blood sugar levels and promote feelings of fullness. Almond milk is low in potassium and phosphorus, making it a great alternative to dairy milk for those with kidney disease. Frozen mixed berries are rich in antioxidants and fibre, while chia seeds and ground flaxseed are excellent sources of omega-3 fatty acids and fibre. Honey (if desired) adds a touch of sweetness without adding too many calories or carbohydrates. Cinnamon and vanilla extract add flavour without adding excess sodium or potassium. Overall, this Berry Blast Oatmeal Bowl is a healthy and satisfying breakfast option that is perfect for those following a diabetic renal diet.

## Spinach and Feta Omelette

Spinach and Feta Omelette is a delicious and nutritious breakfast option that is perfect for those following a diabetic renal diet. This recipe is low in sodium, potassium, and phosphorus, making it a great choice for individuals with kidney disease who are also managing their blood sugar levels.

**Ingredients:**
- 2 large eggs
- 1 cup fresh spinach, chopped
- 2 tablespoons crumbled feta cheese
- 1/4 teaspoon salt-free seasoning blend (such as Mrs. Dash)
- 1 tablespoon olive oil

**Instructions:**
1. In a medium bowl, whisk together the eggs and salt-free seasoning blend. Set aside.
2. Heat the olive oil in a nonstick skillet over medium heat. Add the chopped spinach and sauté for 2-3 minutes, or until wilted.
3. Pour the beaten eggs into the skillet and use a spatula to spread the spinach evenly throughout the eggs.
4. Sprinkle the crumbled feta cheese over the top of the omelette.
5. Cook the omelette for 2-3 minutes on each side, or until set and golden brown.
6. Slide the omelette onto a plate and serve immediately.

This Spinach and Feta Omelette is packed with protein from the eggs and feta cheese, as well as fibre and vitamins from the spinach. It is a satisfying and healthy breakfast option that will keep you

feeling full and energised throughout the morning.
Enjoy!

## Chia Seed Pudding with Fresh Berries

Chia seed pudding is a delicious and healthy breakfast option that is perfect for those following a diabetic renal diet. This recipe is not only low in sugar and sodium, but it's also high in fibre, protein, and essential minerals like calcium and magnesium.

**Ingredients:**
- 1/4 cup chia seeds
- 1 cup unsweetened almond milk (or any non-dairy milk of your choice)
- 1/2 cup fresh berries (such as strawberries, raspberries, and blueberries)
- 1 tablespoon honey (or any natural sweetener of your choice)
- 1/2 teaspoon vanilla extract
- 1/4 teaspoon ground cinnamon

**Instructions:**
1. In a mixing bowl, combine chia seeds, almond milk, honey, vanilla extract, and cinnamon. Stir well until the chia seeds are evenly distributed.
2. Let the mixture sit for at least 30 minutes or overnight in the refrigerator. The chia seeds will absorb the liquid and form a pudding-like texture.a

3. Before serving, gently fold in the fresh berries. This will prevent the berries from breaking down and releasing too much liquid into the pudding.
4. Divide the chia seed pudding into individual serving bowls and enjoy! You can also top it with additional fresh berries or a sprinkle of cinnamon for extra flavor and texture.

This chia seed pudding is not only delicious but also packed with nutrients that are beneficial for people with diabetes and kidney disease. Chia seeds are rich in fibre, which helps to regulate blood sugar levels and promote feelings of fullness, making it a great option for managing diabetes. They're also low in sodium, which is important for people with kidney disease as they need to limit their intake of salt to prevent fluid buildup in their bodies. Additionally, fresh berries are low in sugar and high in antioxidants, which can help to protect against inflammation and oxidative stress, both of which are risk factors for diabetes and kidney disease. Overall, this chia seed pudding is a nutritious and satisfying breakfast option that is easy to prepare and customizable to your taste preferences.

# Low Phosphorus Meats

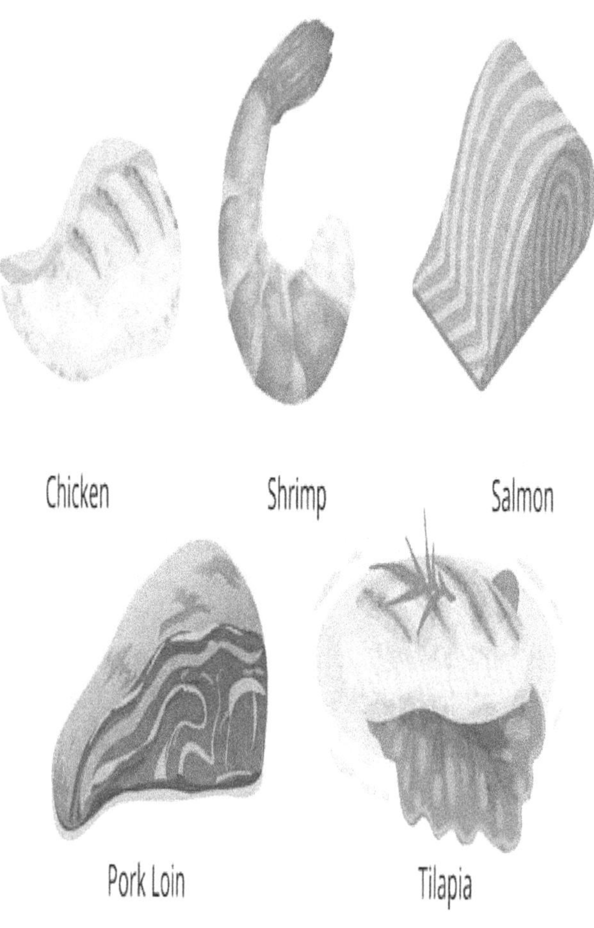

# CHAPTER THREE

## Satisfying Snacks

### Roasted Chickpeas with Herbs

Roasted Chickpeas with Herbs: A Satisfying Snack for Diabetic Renal Diet

If you're following a diabetic renal diet, finding satisfying snacks that are both healthy and delicious can be a challenge. However, roasted chickpeas with herbs are a tasty and nutritious option that are perfect for this diet. Here's how to make them:

**Ingredients:**
- 1 can (15 oz) washed and drained chickpeas
- 1 tbsp olive oil
- 1 tsp dried oregano
- 1 tsp dried basil
- 1 tsp dried thyme
- 1/2 tsp garlic powder
- Salt and pepper to taste

**Instructions:**
1. Preheat your oven to 400°F (200°C).
2. Rinse and drain the chickpeas, then pat them dry with a clean towel or paper towel. This will aid in crisping them up in the oven.

3. In a bowl, mix together the olive oil, oregano, basil, thyme, garlic powder, salt, and pepper. Add the chickpeas and toss until they are evenly coated.
4. Spread the chickpeas out in a single layer on a baking sheet lined with parchment paper. Make sure they are not too crowded, as this will prevent them from getting crispy.
5. Roast the chickpeas in the oven for 20-25 minutes, or until they are golden brown and crispy. To achieve equal roasting, stir them once or twice during cooking.
6. Take the chickpeas out of the oven and set aside for a few minutes before serving.
Enjoy as a satisfying snack that is low in sodium, high in protein and fibre, and packed with flavour!

## Veggie Sticks with Hummus

In a diabetic renal diet, it's essential to choose snacks that are both satisfying and healthy, especially for those with kidney disease. Veggie sticks with hummus are an excellent choice as they provide a good balance of protein, fibre, and healthy fats.

Veggie sticks are low in calories and carbohydrates, making them a perfect snack for people with diabetes. They're also rich in vitamins and minerals, such as vitamin C, potassium, and fibre. Some great veggie options include carrots, celery, cucumber, bell peppers, and cherry tomatoes.

Hummus is a dip made from chickpeas, tahini (sesame seed paste), olive oil, lemon juice, and garlic. It's an excellent source of plant-based protein and healthy fats that help keep you full for longer. Hummus is also low in sodium and potassium, making it a suitable choice for people with kidney disease.

To make veggie sticks with hummus at home, you can either buy pre-made hummus or make your own using a food processor or blender. Here's a simple recipe:

**Ingredients:**
- 1 can (15 oz) washed and drained chickpeas
- 2 cloves garlic
- 2 tbsp tahini
- 2 tbsp lemon juice
- 2 tbsp olive oil
- Salt and pepper to taste
- Water (optional)

**Instructions:**
1. Add the chickpeas, garlic, tahini, lemon juice, and olive oil to a food processor or blender. Blend until smooth.
2. Season with salt and pepper to taste. If the hummus is too thick, add water a tablespoon at a time until you reach the desired consistency.

3. Transfer the hummus to a serving dish and refrigerate for at least 30 minutes before serving. This will allow the flavours to meld together.
4. Serve with your favourite veggie sticks and enjoy!

In summary, veggie sticks with hummus are an excellent choice for satisfying snacks in a diabetic renal diet cookbook for beginners as they're low in calories and carbohydrates, rich in nutrients, and provide a good balance of protein, fibre, and healthy fats. Give this recipe a try and experiment with different veggies to find your favourite combination!

## Nutty Trail Mix for On-the-Go Energy

A Perfect Snack for On-the-Go Energy in Diabetic Renal Diet Cookbook for Beginners

When it comes to satisfying snacks that provide a quick burst of energy, it's hard to beat the convenience and nutritional benefits of nutty trail mix. This delicious and healthy snack is an excellent choice for individuals following a diabetic renal diet, as it is low in sodium, sugar, and potassium while still packing a punch of protein and healthy fats.

Here's how to make your own nutty trail mix that is both delicious and diabetic renal diet-friendly:

**Ingredients:**
- 1/2 cup unsalted almonds
- 1/2 cup unsalted cashews
- 1/4 cup unsalted pumpkin seeds
- 1/4 cup unsalted sunflower seeds
- 1/4 cup unsweetened dried cranberries
- 1/4 cup unsweetened dried apricots (chopped)
- 1/4 cup unsweetened dried cherries (chopped)
- 1/4 cup unsweetened shredded coconut
- 1 tablespoon chia seeds (optional)

**Instructions:**
1. Rinse all nuts and seeds thoroughly under running water to remove any impurities or excess salt. Pat dry with a clean towel.
2. In a large mixing bowl, combine the almonds, cashews, pumpkin seeds, sunflower seeds, dried cranberries, dried apricots, dried cherries, shredded coconut, and chia seeds (if using). Mix until all of the ingredients are uniformly distributed.
3. Store the trail mix in an airtight container in a cool, dry place. It can be stored for up to two weeks.
4. When ready to eat, portion out a serving size of approximately 1/4 cup (about 40 grams) and enjoy it as a satisfying snack on the go! This serving size provides approximately 150 calories, 6 grams of protein, and 8 grams of healthy fats. It is also low in sodium (less than 5 milligrams per serving), sugar (less than 5 grams per serving), and potassium (less than 200 milligrams per serving).

5. For added convenience, you can also pack individual portions of trail mix in small resealable bags or containers for easy transport in your purse, backpack, or car. This makes it easy to grab a quick snack whenever you need a boost of energy throughout the day!

# CHAPTER FOUR

## Wholesome Lunches

### Quinoa and Grilled Vegetable Salad

Quinoa and Grilled Vegetable Salad is a delicious and nutritious option for those following a diabetic renal diet. This recipe is perfect for wholesome lunches as it is low in sodium, potassium, and phosphorus, making it suitable for individuals with kidney disease.

**Ingredients:**
- 1 cup quinoa, rinsed
- 2 cups water
- 1 red bell pepper, sliced
- 1 yellow bell pepper, sliced
- 1 zucchini, sliced
- 1 red onion, sliced
- 2 tablespoons olive oil
- 2 tablespoons balsamic vinegar
- 1 tablespoon lemon juice
- Salt and pepper to taste
- Optional garnish of fresh parsley or cilantro

**Instructions:**

1. Preheat the grill to medium-high heat. Brush the bell peppers, zucchini, and red onion with olive oil and season with salt and pepper. Grill the

vegetables for 3-4 minutes per side or until tender and lightly charred. Set aside.

2. Rinse the quinoa thoroughly in cold water to remove any bitterness. In a medium saucepan, combine the quinoa and water. Bring to a boil over high heat. Reduce heat to low and simmer for 15-20 minutes or until the water is absorbed and the quinoa is tender. Set aside after fluffing with a fork.

3. In a small bowl, whisk together the olive oil, balsamic vinegar, and lemon juice to make the dressing. Season with salt and pepper to taste.

4. In a large mixing bowl, combine the grilled vegetables and cooked quinoa. Toss the salad lightly with the dressing to mix. If preferred, garnish with fresh parsley or cilantro. Refrigerate until ready to serve or serve immediately. Enjoy your wholesome lunch!

## Lemon Garlic Baked Salmon

Lemon Garlic Baked Salmon is a delicious and healthy option for those following a diabetic renal diet. This recipe is low in sodium, potassium, and phosphorus, making it a great choice for individuals with kidney disease who need to manage their intake of these nutrients.

**Ingredients:**
- 4 (6-ounce) salmon fillets
- 2 tablespoons olive oil
- 4 cloves garlic, minced
- 1/4 cup fresh lemon juice
- 1 tablespoon chopped fresh parsley
- Salt and pepper, to taste

**Instructions:**
1. Preheat the oven to 375°F (190°C). Using parchment paper, line a baking dish.
2. Rinse the salmon fillets under cold water and pat them dry with paper towels. Place them in the prepared baking dish.
3. In a small bowl, whisk together the olive oil, garlic, lemon juice, parsley, salt, and pepper. Mixture should be poured over salmon fillets.
4. Bake the salmon for 12-15 minutes or until it is cooked through and flakes easily with a fork.
5. Serve the Lemon Garlic Baked Salmon hot with steamed vegetables and brown rice for a wholesome lunch that is both delicious and nutritious. Enjoy!

## Lentil and Vegetable Soup

Lentil and Vegetable Soup is a delicious and nutritious option for those following a diabetic renal diet. This soup is packed with protein, fibre, and essential vitamins and minerals, making it a wholesome choice for lunch.

**Ingredients:**
- 1 cup brown lentils, rinsed and drained
- 1 onion, chopped
- 2 garlic cloves, minced
- 2 celery stalks, chopped
- 2 carrots, chopped
- 1 red bell pepper, chopped
- 1 can (14.5 oz) undrained diced tomatoes
- 4 cups low-sodium vegetable broth
- 1 tsp dried thyme
- 1 tsp dried oregano
- Salt and pepper to taste
- Fresh parsley for garnish (optional)

**Instructions:**
1. In a large pot, sauté the onion and garlic over medium heat until softened.
2. Add the celery, carrots, and red bell pepper to the pot and cook for another 5 minutes.
3. Add the lentils, diced tomatoes (with juice), vegetable broth, thyme, and oregano to the pot. Stir well.
4. Bring the soup to a boil, then reduce heat to low and simmer for 30-35 minutes or until the lentils are tender.
5. Season with salt and pepper to taste. Garnish with fresh parsley if desired.
6. Serve hot and enjoy your wholesome lunch!

This Lentil and Vegetable Soup is not only delicious but also low in sodium, potassium, and phosphorus

- making it an ideal choice for those with diabetic renal diet restrictions. The high fibre content of lentils also helps regulate blood sugar levels while promoting feelings of fullness. Enjoy this soup as part of a balanced diabetic renal diet meal plan for optimal health benefits!

# Diet Tips For People With Diabetes and Kidney Disease

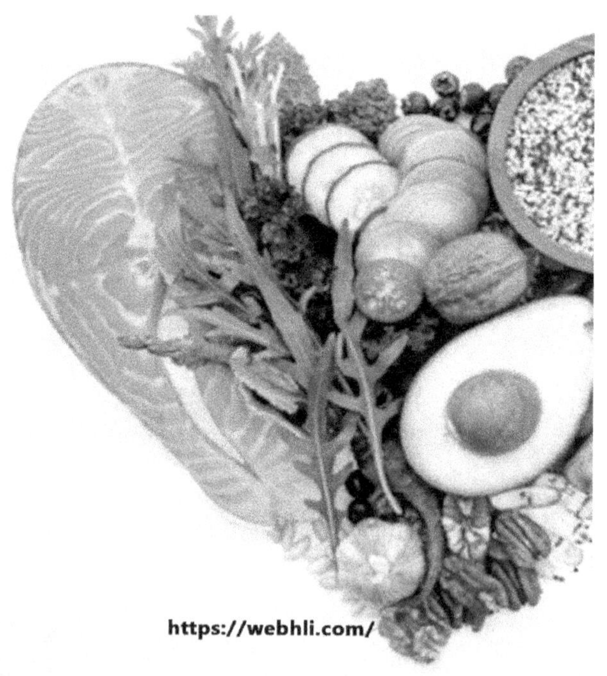

# CHAPTER FIVE

## Flavorful Dinners

### Grilled Chicken with Mediterranean Quinoa

Grilled Chicken with Mediterranean Quinoa is a delicious and healthy meal that is perfect for those following a diabetic renal diet. This dish is packed with flavour and nutrients that will satisfy your taste buds while also supporting your health goals.

The grilled chicken is seasoned with a blend of Mediterranean herbs and spices, including oregano, thyme, and garlic. These flavours add depth and complexity to the chicken, making it both savoury and satisfying. The chicken is also grilled to perfection, ensuring that it is juicy and tender on the inside while crispy on the outside.

The Mediterranean quinoa is a nutritious side dish that complements the chicken perfectly. Quinoa is a complete protein, making it an excellent choice for those following a vegetarian or vegan diet. It is also rich in fibre, which helps to regulate blood sugar levels and promote healthy digestion. The quinoa is cooked with a variety of Mediterranean ingredients, including cherry tomatoes, cucumber, red onion, and Kalamata olives. These ingredients add texture and flavour to the quinoa, making it both refreshing and satisfying.

This dish is low in sodium and potassium, making it an excellent choice for those following a diabetic renal diet. It is also high in protein and fibre, which will help to keep you feeling full and satisfied for longer periods of time. Additionally, this dish is low in carbohydrates, making it a great option for those looking to manage their blood sugar levels.

Here's how to prepare Grilled Chicken with Mediterranean Quinoa:

**Ingredients:**
- 4 boneless, skinless chicken breasts
- 1 tablespoon dried oregano
- 1 tablespoon dried thyme
- 2 cloves garlic, minced
- Salt and pepper to taste
- 1 cup quinoa, rinsed and drained
- 2 cups low-sodium chicken broth
- 1 cup cherry tomatoes, halved
- 1 small cucumber, diced
- 1/4 red onion, diced
- 1/4 cup pitted and chopped Kalamata olives
- 2 tablespoons extra-virgin olive oil
- 2 tablespoons lemon juice
- Fresh parsley for garnish (optional)

**Instructions:**
1. Preheat the grill to medium-high heat. Season chicken breasts with oregano, thyme, garlic, salt, and pepper on both sides. Grill chicken for 6-8 minutes per side or until internal temperature reaches 165°F (74°C). Allow for a 5-minute rest before chopping into strips.
2. In a medium saucepan, combine quinoa and chicken broth. Bring to a boil over high heat. Reduce heat to low and simmer for 15-20 minutes or until quinoa is tender and liquid has been absorbed. Fluff with a fork.
3. In a large mixing bowl, combine cooked quinoa, cherry tomatoes, cucumber, red onion, Kalamata olives, olive oil, lemon juice, salt, and pepper. Toss gently to combine all ingredients evenly. Serve alongside sliced grilled chicken breasts. Garnish with fresh parsley if desired. Enjoy!

## Zucchini Noodles with Pesto and Cherry Tomatoes

Zucchini noodles, also known as zoodles, have become a popular alternative to traditional pasta for those looking for a low-carb and healthier option. They are also a great choice for individuals following a diabetic renal diet, as they are low in calories, carbohydrates, and sodium. In this recipe, we'll be pairing zucchini noodles with a delicious pesto sauce and cherry tomatoes for a flavourful and nutritious dinner that's perfect for beginners following a diabetic renal diet.

**Ingredients:**
- 4 medium-sized zucchinis
- 1/2 cup fresh basil leaves
- 1/4 cup grated Parmesan cheese
- 1/4 cup extra-virgin olive oil
- 2 garlic cloves, peeled
- 1/4 cup pine nuts (optional)
- Salt and pepper to taste
- 1 pint cherry tomatoes, halved

**Instructions:**
1. Begin by washing the zucchinis thoroughly and trimming off the ends. Use a spiralizer or vegetable peeler to create long, thin noodles from the zucchinis. Set aside.
2. In a food processor or blender, combine the basil leaves, Parmesan cheese, olive oil, garlic cloves, and pine nuts (if using). Pulse the contents until they are finely minced and well blended. Season with salt and pepper to taste.
3. In a large skillet over medium heat, sauté the cherry tomatoes until they are slightly softened and lightly browned. Remove from the skillet and set aside.
4. Add the zucchini noodles to the same skillet and sauté for 2-3 minutes until they are slightly tender but still crisp. Remove from heat.
5. Add the pesto sauce to the skillet with the zucchini noodles and toss until the noodles are evenly coated with the sauce. Add the sautéed

cherry tomatoes back into the skillet and toss again to combine all ingredients.

6. Serve hot and enjoy your delicious and healthy diabetic renal diet dinner! This recipe makes approximately 4 servings, each containing approximately 150 calories, 8 grams of carbohydrates, 6 grams of protein, and 12 grams of fat (with pine nuts). If you prefer a lower fat version, you can omit the pine nuts from the pesto sauce or substitute them with walnuts or almonds instead.

## Black Bean and Vegetable Stir-Fry

A Delicious and Healthy Meal for Diabetics with Renal Disease

When it comes to managing diabetes and renal disease, it's essential to follow a specific diet that is low in sodium, potassium, and phosphorus. This recipe for black bean and vegetable stir-fry is not only flavorful but also meets the dietary requirements of diabetics with renal disease.

**Ingredients:**
- 1 can (15 oz) rinsed and drained black beans
- 1 red bell pepper, sliced
- 1 yellow bell pepper, sliced
- 1 small onion, diced
- 2 garlic cloves, minced
- 1 tbsp olive oil
- 1 tbsp low sodium soy sauce
- 1 tsp dried oregano

- 1 tsp dried thyme
- Salt and pepper to taste
- Lemon wedges for garnish (optional)

**Instructions:**
1. Heat olive oil in a large skillet over medium heat. Sauté the garlic and onion for 2-3 minutes, or until aromatic.
2. Add bell peppers and cook for another 5 minutes until they are tender.
3. Add black beans, soy sauce, oregano, thyme, salt, and pepper. Stir everything together thoroughly.
4. Cook for another 2-3 minutes until the vegetables are heated through.
5. Serve hot with lemon wedges on the side (optional).

This black bean and vegetable stir-fry is an excellent source of protein, fibre, and essential vitamins and minerals that are beneficial for diabetics with renal disease. Black beans are low in sodium and potassium but high in protein, making them an excellent alternative to meat. Bell peppers are rich in vitamin C, while onions contain antioxidants that help reduce inflammation. Garlic adds flavour without adding excess sodium or potassium. This dish is also low in phosphorus, making it a perfect choice for individuals with renal disease who need to limit their phosphorus intake. Enjoy this flavorful and healthy meal as part of your diabetic renal diet!

# CHAPTER SIX

## Sweet Endings

### Mixed Berry Parfait

Mixed Berry Parfait is the perfect sweet ending for those following a diabetic renal diet. This delicious and healthy dessert is packed with flavorful berries, creamy yoghurt, and crunchy granola, making it a satisfying treat that won't spike your blood sugar levels.

**Ingredients:**
- 1 cup fresh strawberries, sliced
- 1 cup fresh blueberries
- 1 cup fresh raspberries
- 1 cup plain low-fat Greek yoghourt
- 1/2 cup granola (make sure it's low in sodium and sugar)

**Instructions:**
1. Wash and slice the strawberries.
2. Rinse the blueberries and raspberries.
3. In four separate glasses, layer the berries and yoghurt, starting with the berries at the bottom.
4. Sprinkle a generous amount of granola on top of each parfait.

5. Serve immediately and enjoy!

This mixed berry parfait is not only delicious but also rich in fibre, vitamins, and minerals that are essential for people with diabetes and kidney disease. The low-fat Greek yoghurt is a great source of protein, while the berries are packed with antioxidants and fibre that help regulate blood sugar levels. The granola adds a crunchy texture and provides healthy fats and fibre to keep you feeling full and satisfied.

When following a diabetic renal diet, it's essential to choose foods that are low in sodium, potassium, and phosphorus to prevent further damage to your kidneys. This mixed berry parfait is a perfect dessert option as it meets these dietary requirements while still being delicious and satisfying. It's also easy to prepare and can be made ahead of time for a quick and healthy sweet treat anytime you want!

## Avocado Chocolate Mousse

Avocado Chocolate Mousse is a delicious and healthy dessert option for those following a diabetic renal diet. This recipe is low in sugar, salt, and potassium, making it a perfect choice for individuals with diabetes and kidney disease.

**Ingredients:**
- 2 ripe avocados

- 1/4 cup unsweetened cocoa powder
- 1/4 cup almond milk
- 1/4 cup unsweetened applesauce
- 1/4 cup Stevia (or other sugar substitute)
- 1 tsp vanilla extract
- 1 tsp lemon juice

**Instructions:**
1. Halve the avocados and remove the pit. Scoop out the flesh and toss it in a food processor or blender.
2. Add the cocoa powder, almond milk, applesauce, Stevia, vanilla extract, and lemon juice to the blender.
3. Blend all the ingredients until they are smooth and creamy. If the mixture is too thick, you can add a little more almond milk to thin it out.
4. Divide the mousse into four small bowls or ramekins.
5. Chill the mousse in the refrigerator for at least 30 minutes before serving to allow it to set.
6. Serve chilled and enjoy your healthy and delicious Avocado Chocolate Mousse!

This recipe is low in sugar, salt, and potassium, making it a great option for individuals with diabetes and kidney disease. Avocados are a good source of healthy fats, fibre, and potassium, while cocoa powder is rich in antioxidants. Almond milk is low in calories and fat, making it a healthier alternative to traditional dairy products. Applesauce adds natural sweetness without adding excess sugar or calories.

Stevia is a sugar substitute that is low in calories and does not affect blood sugar levels like regular sugar does. Lemon juice helps to balance the flavours and adds a tangy twist to the mousse. This recipe is not only delicious but also nutritious and easy to prepare!

## Baked Apple Slices with Cinnamon

A Delicious and Healthy Dessert for Diabetics on a Renal Diet

If you're a diabetic on a renal diet, you may think that satisfying your sweet tooth is impossible. However, with a little creativity, you can enjoy delicious desserts that are both healthy and low in sugar and sodium. In this recipe, we'll show you how to make baked apple slices with cinnamon, a simple and tasty dessert that's perfect for those following a diabetic renal diet.

**Ingredients:**
- 2 medium apples (Granny Smith or Honeycrisp)
- 1 tablespoon lemon juice
- 1 teaspoon ground cinnamon
- 1 tablespoon unsalted butter, melted
- 1 tablespoon honey (optional)

**Instructions:**

1. Preheat your oven to 375°F (190°C). Using parchment paper, line a baking sheet.

2. Wash the apples and remove the core and seeds. Cut the apples into thin slices, about ¼ inch thick. Put the slices in a large mixing basin.

3. Add lemon juice to the bowl with the apple slices. This will prevent them from browning and add a tangy flavor. Mix well.

4. Sprinkle cinnamon over the apple slices and toss gently to coat evenly.

5. In a small saucepan over low heat, melt the butter. Add honey (if using) and mix well. Pour the mixture over the apple slices and toss again to coat evenly.

6. Arrange the apple slices in a single layer on the prepared baking sheet, making sure they don't overlap. Bake for 15-20 minutes or until the apples are tender and lightly browned around the edges.

7. Remove from the oven and set aside for a few minutes to cool before serving. You can serve them warm or at room temperature, garnished with additional cinnamon if desired. Enjoy your baked apple slices as a healthy and satisfying dessert!

**Nutrition Information (per serving):**
Calories: 80 | Total Fat: 3g | Saturated Fat: 2g | Cholesterol: 8mg | Sodium: 3mg | Total

Carbohydrate: 13g | Dietary Fibre: 3g | Total
Sugars: 9g (including 6g added sugars)
| Protein: 1g | Potassium: 140mg
| Phosphorus: 20mg | Calcium: 4mg
| Vitamin C: 4mg | Iron: 0mg
| Magnesium: 15mg | Zinc: 0mg | Copper: 0mg
| Manganese: 0mg
| Vitamin A IU: 45IU | Vitamin E IU: 0IU
| Vitamin K IU: 2IU | Thiamin IU: 0IU
| Riboflavin IU: 0IU | Niacin IU: 1 IU
| Folate DFE IU: 9 mcg DFE | Vitamin B12 IU: 0IU |
Pantothenic Acid IU: 0IU

# CHAPTER SEVEN

## Beverages for Wellness

### Citrus Infused Water

A Refreshing and Healthy Beverage for Diabetic Renal Diet

In a world where sugary drinks and high-calorie beverages are easily accessible, it's essential to make healthier choices, especially for those with diabetes and renal issues. Citrus infused water is a simple and delicious way to stay hydrated while also providing numerous health benefits. In this article, we'll explore the benefits of citrus infused water for diabetics following a renal diet and provide some easy-to-follow recipes.

Benefits of Citrus Infused Water for Diabetics on a Renal Diet

*1. Low in Calories and Sugar:*

Citrus fruits like lemons, limes, oranges, and grapefruits are naturally low in calories and sugar. By infusing water with these fruits, you can create a refreshing beverage that's low in calories and sugar, making it an excellent choice for diabetics following a renal diet.

*2. Rich in Vitamins and Minerals:*

Citrus fruits are packed with vitamins and minerals that are essential for overall health. For instance, lemons are rich in vitamin C, which helps boost the immune system, while oranges are a good source of potassium, which is important for maintaining healthy blood pressure.

*3. Promotes Hydration:*

Staying hydrated is crucial for individuals with diabetes and renal issues as it helps prevent dehydration, which can lead to complications such as kidney stones. Infusing water with citrus fruits adds flavour to the water, making it more appealing to drink, which can help increase water intake throughout the day.

*4. Helps Regulate Blood Sugar:*

Citrus fruits contain fibre, which helps slow down the absorption of sugar into the bloodstream. This can help regulate blood sugar levels in individuals with diabetes.

Easy Citrus Infused Water Recipes for Diabetics on a Renal Diet

**1. Lemon-Mint Infused Water:** Slice a lemon into thin rounds and add them to a pitcher of water along with a handful of fresh mint leaves. Let it sit in the refrigerator for at least 2 hours before serving to allow the flavours to infuse into the water.

**2. Orange-Cinnamon Infused Water:** Peel an orange using a vegetable peeler to remove the zest (avoiding the white pith) and add it to a pitcher of water along with a cinnamon stick. Allow it to chill for at least 2 hours before serving.

**3. Grapefruit-Rosemary Infused Water:** Slice a grapefruit into thin rounds and add them to a pitcher of water along with a few sprigs of fresh rosemary. Allow it to chill for at least 2 hours before serving.

In conclusion, citrus infused water is an excellent choice for diabetics following a renal diet as it's low in calories and sugar, rich in vitamins and minerals, promotes hydration, and helps regulate blood sugar levels. By following our easy citrus infused water recipes, you can create delicious and healthy beverages that will keep you hydrated throughout the day while also providing numerous health benefits.

## Herbal Tea Blends for Kidney Support

Herbal tea blends have gained popularity in recent years as a natural and healthy alternative to traditional caffeinated beverages. For individuals with diabetes and kidney issues, herbal teas can offer a variety of benefits, including supporting kidney function and promoting overall wellness. In this article, we will explore some herbal tea blends that are particularly beneficial for kidney support and provide tips on how to incorporate them into a diabetic renal diet cookbook for beginners.

## 1. Dandelion Root Tea

Dandelion root tea is a popular choice for kidney support due to its diuretic properties. It helps to increase urine output, which can help to flush out excess fluid and toxins from the body. Dandelion root tea is also rich in antioxidants, which can help to protect the kidneys from damage caused by free radicals. To prepare dandelion root tea, steep 1-2 teaspoons of dried dandelion root in hot water for 10-15 minutes.

## 2. Nettle Leaf Tea

Nettle leaf tea is another herbal tea that is beneficial for kidney health. It contains compounds that can help to prevent the formation of kidney stones and reduce inflammation in the urinary tract. Nettle leaf tea is also rich in vitamins and minerals, including vitamin C, iron, and calcium. To prepare nettle leaf tea, steep 1-2 teaspoons of dried nettle leaves in hot water for 10-15 minutes.

## 3. Marshmallow Root Tea

Marshmallow root tea has a soothing effect on the urinary tract and can help to alleviate symptoms of urinary tract infections (UTIs). It also contains compounds that can help to reduce inflammation in the kidneys. Marshmallow root tea is sweet and mellow, making it a pleasant option for those who prefer a less bitter taste. To prepare marshmallow root tea, steep 1-2 teaspoons of dried marshmallow root in hot water for 10-15 minutes.

4. Juniper Berry Tea

Juniper berry tea has been used traditionally as a diuretic and to promote kidney health. It contains compounds that can help to prevent the formation of kidney stones and reduce inflammation in the urinary tract. Juniper berry tea also has a pleasant aroma and flavour, making it an enjoyable option for those who prefer a more complex taste profile. To prepare juniper berry tea, steep 1-2 teaspoons of dried juniper berries in hot water for 10-15 minutes.

Incorporating Herbal Tea Blends into a Diabetic Renal Diet Cookbook for Beginners:

Here are some tips on how to incorporate herbal tea blends into a diabetic renal diet cookbook for beginners:

- Choose low-sodium options: If you have diabetes and kidney issues, it's important to choose herbal teas that are low in sodium to help manage blood pressure levels. Look for teas that are labelled "low sodium" or "no salt added."

- Limit caffeine: Caffeine can increase blood sugar levels and dehydrate the body, which can put additional strain on the kidneys. Choose herbal teas that are naturally caffeine-free or contain very low amounts of caffeine.

- Watch out for added sugars: Some herbal teas may contain added sugars or sweeteners, which can increase blood sugar levels and contribute to weight gain. Choose unsweetened options or use natural sweeteners like stevia or honey in moderation.

- Experiment with blends: Don't be afraid to mix and match different herbal teas to create your own unique blends! Combining dandelion root, nettle leaf, marshmallow root, and juniper berry teas can create a delicious and well-rounded blend that supports overall kidney health and wellness.

In conclusion, incorporating herbal tea blends into a diabetic renal diet cookbook for beginners can offer numerous benefits for kidney health and overall wellness. By choosing low-sodium options, limiting caffeine, watching out for added sugars, and experimenting with blends, you can create delicious and healthy beverages that support your unique needs as someone with diabetes and kidney issues.

## Refreshing Cucumber Mint Smoothie

In our Diabetic Renal Diet Cookbook for Beginners, we believe that wellness is not just about eating the right foods, but also nourishing our bodies with beverages that are both refreshing and beneficial for our health. One such beverage that perfectly aligns with this philosophy is the Refreshing Cucumber Mint Smoothie.

This smoothie is not only delicious, but also packed with ingredients that offer a multitude of benefits for individuals following a diabetic renal diet.
Let's take a deeper look at the main elements:

**1. Cucumbers:** Cucumbers are incredibly hydrating and low in carbohydrates, making them an ideal ingredient for diabetic individuals. They are also known for their anti-inflammatory properties, promoting overall kidney health.

**2. Mint:** Mint adds a refreshing burst of flavour to this smoothie. It aids in digestion, reduces inflammation, and may help relieve symptoms of indigestion, making it beneficial for those with kidney issues.

**3. Spinach:** Although spinach may seem unconventional in a beverage, it adds a plethora of nutrients without significantly impacting blood sugar levels. It is an excellent source of vitamins A and C and contains minerals like iron and magnesium, promoting overall wellness.

**4. Almond Milk:** As an alternative to traditional dairy milk, almond milk is low in sugar and carbohydrates, making it suitable for individuals with diabetes. It provides a creamy texture to the smoothie without causing an excessive rise in blood glucose levels.

**5. Avocado:** Avocados provide healthy fats that are good for maintaining cardiovascular health. They are low in carbohydrates and high in fibre, promoting a steady release of glucose into the bloodstream.

To prepare this Refreshing Cucumber Mint Smoothie, simply combine sliced cucumbers, fresh mint leaves, a handful of spinach, a dash of almond milk, and half an avocado in a blender. Blend until smooth and creamy, adding ice cubes if desired. This smoothie can be enjoyed as a refreshing beverage or as a light meal option for those following a diabetic renal diet.

At our Diabetic Renal Diet Cookbook for Beginners, we believe that beverages should not only taste great but also contribute to overall wellness. The

Refreshing Cucumber Mint Smoothie is a perfect addition to our collection of recipes, offering a refreshing and nourishing option for individuals striving for optimal health even within dietary restrictions.

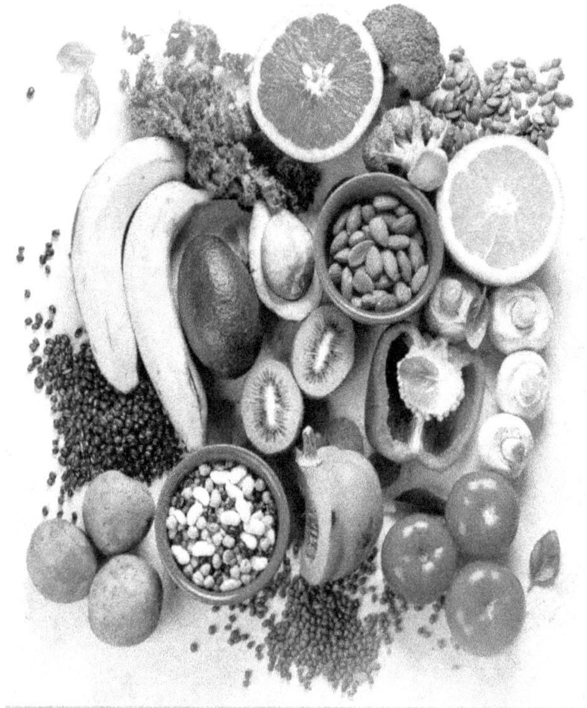

THE LOW-POTASSIUM DIET
What You Need to Know
From a Renal Dietitian
www.PlantPoweredKidneys.com

# CONCLUSION

## Nutritional Information

In a diabetic renal diet, it's crucial to manage both blood sugar and kidney function. For individuals with diabetes and kidney disease, following a specific dietary plan is essential to maintain optimal health. This cookbook for beginners aims to provide delicious and nutritious recipes that cater to the unique nutritional requirements of those with diabetic renal disease.

Here's a breakdown of the nutritional information you'll find in this cookbook:

*1. Calorie Control:*

Diabetic renal disease can lead to weight loss, making it essential to consume enough calories to maintain a healthy weight. However, excessive calorie intake can put additional strain on the kidneys. This cookbook provides recipes that are low in calories but high in nutrients, helping individuals maintain a healthy weight without compromising their kidney health.

*2. Protein Management:*

Protein is essential for building and repairing tissues, but excessive protein intake can put additional strain on the kidneys. This cookbook provides recipes that are low in protein but still provide enough to meet daily requirements. Additionally, it provides information on which types of protein are best for individuals with diabetic renal disease.

### 3. Sodium Restriction:

High sodium intake can lead to fluid retention and increased blood pressure, which can worsen kidney function in individuals with diabetic renal disease. This cookbook provides recipes that are low in sodium, helping individuals manage their fluid intake and blood pressure.

### 4. Potassium Control:

Potassium is essential for maintaining healthy kidney function, but excessive potassium intake can be dangerous for individuals with diabetic renal disease. This cookbook provides recipes that are low in potassium but still provide enough to meet daily requirements. Additionally, it provides information on which types of potassium-rich foods are best for individuals with diabetic renal disease.

### 5. Blood Sugar Management:

Maintaining stable blood sugar levels is crucial for individuals with diabetes, as high blood sugar levels can worsen kidney function. This cookbook provides recipes that are low in sugar and carbohydrates but still provide enough to meet daily requirements. Additionally, it provides information on how to substitute high-carbohydrate ingredients with lower-carbohydrate alternatives.

Also, this cookbook aims to provide delicious and nutritious recipes that cater to the unique nutritional requirements of individuals with diabetic renal disease while managing blood sugar, protein, sodium, and potassium levels. By following this dietary plan, individuals can maintain optimal health and manage their diabetes and kidney disease effectively.

In conclusion, the Diabetic Renal Diet Cookbook for Beginners is an essential resource for individuals with both diabetes and kidney disease. The cookbook provides a comprehensive guide on how to manage these conditions through a healthy and delicious diet. The recipes are not only nutritionally balanced but also flavorful and easy to prepare, making it an ideal choice for those who want to enjoy their meals while adhering to their dietary restrictions. With the help of this cookbook, individuals can take control of their health and improve their overall well-being. It is a must-have resource for anyone looking to maintain a healthy lifestyle while dealing with diabetes and kidney disease.

# Low Potassium Fruits & Veggies

@plant.powered.kidneys

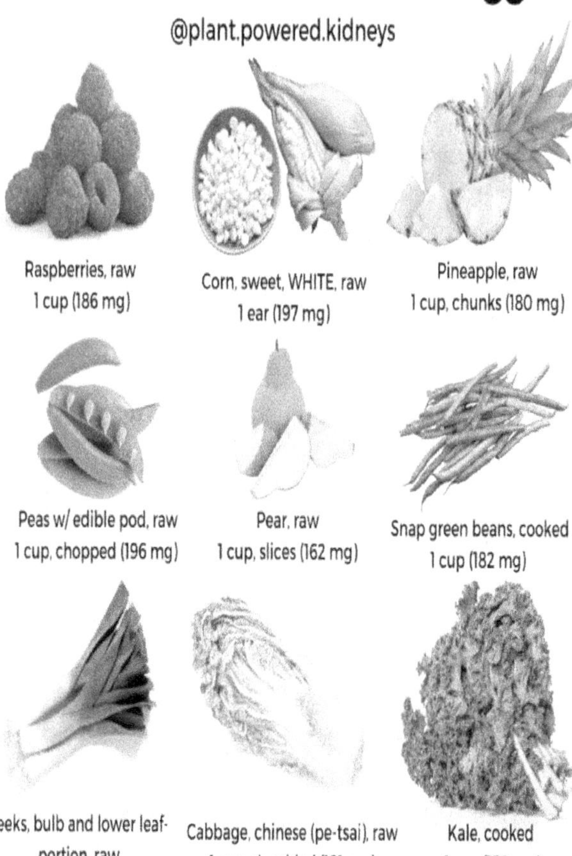

Raspberries, raw
1 cup (186 mg)

Corn, sweet, WHITE, raw
1 ear (197 mg)

Pineapple, raw
1 cup, chunks (180 mg)

Peas w/ edible pod, raw
1 cup, chopped (196 mg)

Pear, raw
1 cup, slices (162 mg)

Snap green beans, cooked
1 cup (182 mg)

Leeks, bulb and lower leaf-
portion, raw
1 cup (160 mg)

Cabbage, chinese (pe-tsai), raw
1 cup, shredded (181 mg)

Kale, cooked
1 cup (170 mg)